GW00481723

NO MEALS AFTER 6:00 P.M.

SERGEANT ZIMMIE WILLIAMS

Los Angeles Police Department

(RET,) FORMER MEMBER OF THE U.S. NAVY

Print ISBN: 978-1-09832-344-8

eBook ISBN: 978-1-09832-345-5

TABLE OF CONTENTS

INTRODUCTION

Fitness is a trait of the strong and healthy; something we all value. Those who are fit—thrive, while those who are not fit sometimes tend to suffer. Those who are not fit suffer from diabetes, heart problems, knee pain, and sometimes back pain as well, caused by carrying extra, excess (undesired) weight. Those who are not fit sometimes suffer from low self-esteem. Why is that so?

Because ever since we were kids, our society has taught us that unless you are "slender, skinny, or thin," you will not be considered attractive.

Through this book I intend to use my service to our country in the United States Navy, and as a Los Angeles police officer and patrol sergeant, to help those who want to step out of a life of "not being fit."

QUESTION: Why are the vast majority of police officers and military members fit?

ANSWER: Because they have to be. Because they are required to be. Because they must be.

QUESTION: Why do people get fat and out of shape?

ANSWER: Because after we leave high school, or college, or the military, we leave the rigidly structured environments that had held us accountable. We leave behind the systems that forced us to conform to a set regime of daily physical exertion. We become overwhelmed by life. Our duties to our jobs and our families take priority. We are so busy watching the clock, ensuring our kids are up and ready for school, ensuring we are dressed and ready for the work environment that we sometimes forget to take time to care for ourselves.

We grow complacent in our obligations, like our duty to make dinner and small talk with the kids and our spouses after a hard day at work or at school. Then, after a satisfying meal, and a few conversational exchanges, we find our way to the television's remote control. We settle in and engage in our favorite pastime; our reward for a long hard day at work and parenting. We watch television. Sometimes, while watching television, we reward ourselves for a hard day at work, and maybe even a difficult time dealing with a supervisor or a subordinate. In an attempt to reward ourselves for a difficult work day, we open the fridge or the kitchen cabinets, and search for something that will make it all better. We search for 'comfort foods and snacks.' Our favorite ice cream, potato chips, blueberry, or cherry pie becomes our salvation and our reward.

After years, or in some cases, just months of doing this, we begin to complain to ourselves that the laundry room dryer or local dry cleaning store has been shrinking our clothes. You avoid the bathroom scale because you secretly know that you have put on 5, 10, 15, 20, or even 30 pounds or more of undesired weight. You know that you've "gained a little weight."

It really isn't that big of a problem until you see yourself in a photograph taken at a family gathering or work event, and you realize the reality of what you've done to yourself.

You tell yourself or your partner, that you really need to get back to the gym, but it will have to wait until the summer, or just after the holidays, or after another artificial line drawn in the sand. Each promised date to tackle the problem comes and goes, while the problem only gets worse.

Then, one day, while you're surfing online, or browsing at a bookstore, or perhaps perusing through a newspaper article, you come across the advertisement of THIS BOOK. You admit to yourself that you're not just a couple of pounds overweight, but that you're "chubby" or "fat."

You say to yourself, "hey, cops are fit; this might be something that can help me." So, you order a copy of this book online; or, if you're in a bookstore, you carry it to the checkout line and purchase it.

The idea of being trained by a retired police officer and military veteran is appealing because of the training this person has been through and completed. The months required to survive "boot camp" and a "police academy" most surely have provided this person with insights that can benefit you in your own quest for physical fitness.

However, the most important lesson that I can impart to you, the reader, is that you must develop a 'mindset' for fitness. You must develop within yourself a desire to change from the 'old you' into the person you want to become. Unless your mind is set on achieving a certain level of personal fitness, all the instruction, books, videos, personal fitness trainers, and coaches in the world will be worthless. Without a developed mindset and a strong desire to achieve and maintain your fitness goal, all of these things are just paper and instruction DVDs that are taking up space in your home, apartment, and gym bag.

A MINDSET:

A mindset for fitness is one that says "I don't care how my day went at work, school, or with my partner, spouse, or the kids, I'm going to take care of myself regardless." It is a mindset that says: "I know the office crew is going out to a nice restaurant with many delicious meal selections that are tempting to me, but because I love myself and I have determined my fitness goal, I will stick to my predetermined diet plan."

It is a mindset that gives you the strength to remove unhealthy items from your home or apartment that tempt you. It pushes you to make time for your workout routine before your workday, or the first class at college, or after you have come home and fulfilled your duties as a partner, and parent. It is a mindset that says no matter what, you will exercise your body and burn the excess calories that caused you to seek out and purchase this book. It is a mindset that causes you to pre-plan the meal you will take to work or school for your lunch break, so that you remain within your desired health and fitness goal.

MILITARY VETERANS AND POLICE OFFICERS HAVE A 'MINDSET':

The reason that military personnel and police officers have a mind-set for fitness is because of the nature of our jobs. Both of these professions are front-line defenders. When the country is forced into a war or a situation where hostilities force aggressive moves, Soldiers, Sailors, Airmen, and Marines don't have the luxury of telling the enemy, "sorry guys, I'm not really ready for war today. Give me two or three months to train, and I will see you on the designated battlefield."

When police officers don their department's uniform, bulletproof vest, weapon, handcuffs, and other required equipment and deploy into the field in a marked black and white (or other color scheme) police vehicle, they don't have the luxury to refuse to provide their services to a citizen by saying that they are not ready for a violent confrontation.

In each of the scenarios listed above, the military service member and the police officer must be fit for duty. For people in the military, that duty could be to march for hours in an effort to reach an objective. Then, once reached, they may be required to engage in a long, protracted battle against a stubborn and well-armed enemy force.

Police officers are often called upon to respond to situations that materialize within a matter of seconds. These situations are often suddenly violent, requiring the officer to engage in a long foot pursuit, adrenaline pumping vehicle pursuit, or physical altercation with a violent person desperate to escape capture by law enforcement officers.

In all of these scenarios, a mindset of superb physical fitness will be of tremendous benefit to the Soldier, Sailor, Airman, Marine, or police officer when called upon to do his or her duty.

CHAPTER 1

DETERMINING YOUR GOAL

After developing a mindset for physical fitness and wellness, you must then determine your goal.

Fitness goals can be broken down into four basic categories:

1. Weight loss

2. Muscle tone

3. Muscular development

4. Development of increased athletic ability

CATERGORY 1. WEIGHT LOSS:

QUESTION: Why do humans desire to lose weight?

Because by losing extra, undesired weight (fat), we can improve our lives and boost our self-esteem.

By losing weight, we can go from the person who can barely touch their shoes when they reach down to tie them, to a person who can get up and go for an extended walk or run effortlessly. The effort it takes to lug around 10, 20, 30, 40, 50, or more pounds of extra body weight can be extremely taxing.

CATERGORY 2. MUSCLE TONE:

Muscle tone is the resistance of a muscle to active or passive stretch, or overall stiffness of the muscle.

CATERGORY 3. MUSCULAR DEVELOPMENT:

Muscular development is the clear indication of muscle mass, density, shape, and function of muscle cells.

This adaptation allows the muscle to meet exercise or function-induced stress.

CATERGORY 4. DEVELOPMENT OF INCREASED ATHLETIC ABILITY:

Increased athletic ability can be attained by achieving an increase in muscular development.

We will delve more into the areas pertaining to muscular development as we progress into this book (in Chapter 17). But for now, we will move into what this book was primarily written to address, which is weight loss using the method I became familiar with many years ago as a young police officer, known as "No Meals After 6:00 P.M."

CHAPTER 2

NO MEALS AFTER 6:00 P.M.

The idea behind the concept of "No Meals After 6:00 P.M." is that you make the decision that you will consume no food of any kind after 6:00 P.M.

This decision entails that not only will you not have a 'full meal', but that you will also not consume snacks, desserts, or beer products of any kind until you're awake after a good night's sleep the following day.

As stated earlier, I became aware of this philosophy while I was still a relatively young police officer.

I thought it was interesting, but not really important to my life, which is why I discarded it and pushed it away into the deepest recesses of my mind.

When my police career came to an end after a very serious neck injury, I was no longer the person who could run for six miles wearing military fatigues and combat boots on a United States Marine Corps obstacle course. I was no longer the person who tried to maintain the superb level of fitness he had so desired ever since his time as a young sailor in the United States Navy.

I could no longer bench press 310 pounds in a gym while lying flat on my back on the bench press machine. I couldn't train in martial arts for an hour each day at home. It almost felt like I was no longer myself.

The person who graduated the Police Academy many years ago, who weighed an extremely fit and trim 165 pounds of solid muscle, no longer existed.

After going through a divorce and no longer being a young man with a wife, I was left to my own devices – and vices.

CHAPTER 3

LAZINESS

Since my beloved police career and married life were behind me, I was no longer required to maintain any level of fitness. Instead, I entered the world of laziness. The world of going out with friends, eating at restaurants, and ordering pizza at home.

I had become a person who would, out of sheer boredom, drive to a fast food location, order a full meal plus dessert at 8:00 or 9:00 P.M. at night, drive back to my home, and consume it in front of the television. I deluded myself into thinking that since I had ordered a diet soda with the gut-busting meal, I was somehow going to win the war against excess weight gain.

I had grown comfortable with a life of leisure and lack of physical exertion.

CHAPTER 4
OBESITY

Like many people who are overweight, I always had a plan to resolve the issue of how I was going to lose five-pounds and get back to my level of super-fitness.

I had excuses for why I could no longer fit into an L-sized shirt or jacket, excuses for why my pants were too tight.

At one point, my body had gained so much weight that I began to simply pull the front zipper area as close as I could get it, and then use my belt as a sort of lasso to keep my pants from falling down.

Because of my laziness, lack of personal discipline, and extremely poor eating habits, I had allowed my fit and trim United States Navy and Los Angeles Police Academy trained, six-foot tall, 165-pound body, to balloon up to happened at a slow pace: 218 became 210 pounds.

I was a total and complete mess!

CHAPTER 5

SHAME

Even though I was in denial about my physical condition, I still had found no way to resolve it.

I tried the all meat diet, I tried rice cakes, I tried eating nothing but chicken or salads, I tried various diet formula drinks that can be found on the shelves of nearly every grocery store. I even tried weight-loss pills, but nothing worked.

The shame began when I was required to renew my driver's license. When the new license was mailed to my home, I compared the image to the older license that was still in my wallet. The proof of my obesity reflected clearly in the new image. I was nearly unrecognizable.

When I saw how truly fat and bloated my body had become, I felt embarrassed to even be seen in public. I was ashamed when birthdays and other public gatherings required me to leave my home to socialize with people whom I had known for years.

CHAPTER 6

RESOLUTION OF OBESITY PROBLEM

While writing my first book, *Surviving The Oral Interview: Boot Camp For The Mind*, I decided that it was time to do something about the monster that had taken over my life—unhealthy eating, unhealthy living, and obesity.

So, as a brand new writer, I researched the mechanics of authoring a book. I learned that the typical author usually takes between four months to roughly a year to complete a book before it is shipped off to the publisher. My battle plan was to write for roughly seven to eight hours each day, six days a week, taking an hour-long lunch break at the halfway point.

I also decided that it might be a good idea to dust off some of the home gym fitness equipment I had amassed while working as a police officer and patrol sergeant.

While toiling away on my laptop computer, writing my first book, I would steal little breaks to walk on the treadmill or ride one of the two stationary bikes I have in my home.

However, even the addition of exercise was not enough to make a significant difference in my weight problem, until I wrote the section in the book pertaining to not eating anything after 6:00 P.M. I reasoned that if this method of weight management was good enough for the readers of my book, then it was most certainly good enough for me as well.

CHAPTER 7

WEIGHT LOSS

I would begin each day with a very small breakfast; a bowl of hot oat meal, a commercially sold weight loss drink, or some other small, healthy, nutritious meal. But with one change, I would no longer consume any food (of any kind) after 6:00 P.M.

A POUND OF FAT:

According to medical experts, it takes 3,500 calories to create one pound of fat. This also means that it takes a reduction of at least 3,500 calories over the course of one week, two weeks, or a month to eliminate one pound of fat.

SUCCESS:

A book I had allotted five months to write, (*Surviving The Oral Interview: Boot Camp For The Mind*) was completed in nineteen days. I then spent the next two months tearing it apart. I rewrote the 148-page book forty separate times. There were at least 300 spelling mistakes and other grammatical errors that needed to be corrected before it could be sent to the publisher for development. While doing the rewrite of my first book, I began to notice a change in my body.

By not eating anything from 6:00 P.M. to 9:00 A.M., I was depriving my body of any food intake for 15 whole hours, seven days a week.

The initial weight loss happened at a slow place. 218 pounds became 210 pounds, which ultimately became 200 pounds. I knew I was onto something big when my weight dropped to 195 pounds—a body weight status I had not seen in 30 years.

By the time my weight dropped down to 190 pounds, I began posting my progress on Facebook so that my family and friends could revel in my success.

It was when I posted that I was down to 185 pounds that I started getting private messages on Facebook from people who were interested in learning about what I was doing.

The private messages were from fellow police officers and civilians from all over the country.

People were interested in learning how I lost 36 pounds of unwanted fat while writing my first book, The interest expressed by those folks, is what prompted me to write this book.

CHAPTER 8

AN EMPTY STOMACH (KETOSIS)

When we don't consume food after 6:00 P.M., our body reaches a natural state known as ketosis. When we are in ketosis, our body begins to consume fat. This state is reached because the stomach has been completely emptied roughly six to eight hours after your last meal has been consumed.

While in ketosis, the body begins to search for fuel to burn. Since the stomach has been emptied, it turns to food that was previously consumed and is now stored, this food is basically fat. If we consume our last meal at 6:00 P.M., our stomachs should be emptied by natural digestive processes by either midnight or 2:00 A.M.

Once our stomach is empty by 2:00 A.M., the body then has seven full hours to process and burn fat until you once again consume a meal at 9:00 A.M.

This is why "No Meals After 6:00 P.M." is so effective in weight loss or ketosis.

CHAPTER 9

WRITING A SECOND BOOK

Since I'd received such a positive response regarding my weight loss journey on Facebook, I decided to share this weight loss method with the world.

Most people who are overweight feel a sense of shame.

The 700 or so friends and family I have on Facebook are mostly active duty police officers, retired police officers, active duty military types, or civilians I have known for years. Police officers and military people are proud professionals, which is what makes them feel ashamed of any excess weight they could be carrying. Therefore, instead of making public proclamations of their weight loss achievements, they communicated their success stories with me privately.

They told me how "No Meals After 6:00 P.M." has changed their lives. They have gushed about how they have tried one weight loss program after another through the years, and that these programs or diets have failed to produce any real, true weight reduction.

The stories of people I love and care about telling me how this method has resulted in weight loss for them was extremely motivating and fulfilling.

I wrote this book because this method of weight loss, control, and management works. It truly does!

Using the techniques mentioned in the book, I personally lost 36 pounds of excess fat in just six months.

CHAPTER 10

FINANCIAL BENEFITS OF "NO MEALS AFTER 6:00 P.M."

One of the clearly discernable benefits of using this weight loss method is the fact that you will be eating a lot less food.

> NOTE: Because you are no longer leaving the house
> to go through a drive-through window at a popular
> pizza, hamburger, or fast food restaurant, you will no
> longer be spending $50 to $60 dollars per week (like
> I was) trying to numb yourself with food as a distrac-
> tion from your life's problems.

If you maintain this method of calorie intake discipline as a weight management program or lifestyle, you can save nearly $350 or more within six months.

CHAPTER 11

CHEAT DAY

I give all the people I have trained in my home or online what is known as a "cheat day."

Cheat day is one day each week (usually on Sundays for me) when we are allowed to eat pretty much anything we want. (Note: Within reason of course.)

Cheat day is, therefore, a break from the "No Meals After 6:00 P.M." diet routine.

Dieting is hard. While dieting, we deprive ourselves of the things we enjoy eating for pleasure: such as pizza, cake, ice cream, pie, donuts, pastries, and all the other stuff that if consumed at will throughout the day, every day, will, over time, make us fat.

CHAPTER 12

EXERCISE

Exercise is an extremely important component of weight loss. If you have a fitness problem or weight problem, you need to get moving. Our bodies were designed to move. Movement is life, whereas a stagnant, sedentary lifestyle may lead to the development of weight problems, which could eventually lead to a premature death.

Exercise is movement. Movement often means forcing yourself to get up from the sofa and engaging in a physical activity.

Exertion for a prolonged period of time causes the heart muscle to pump more blood through the cardiovascular system.

Exertion causes the various muscle groups to push and pull, stand and walk, and walk and or run.

Exertion means that instead of sitting in front of the TV after the evening meal, you will turn it off, walk into the home gym, or exit your residence, and take in fresh clean air as you tour your neighborhood on foot.

Exercise is making a conscious decision to maintain the biological machine that is your body; the only body you have, and the only body you will ever have.

CHAPTER 13

WALKING

Before beginning a new walking routine, you should invest time in researching the kind of shoes that are best suited for your outdoor or treadmill activities.

You should choose shoes that offer comfort, support, and a price that fits within your budget.

Once you have selected shoes that are appropriate for this type of activity, you should next decide on when you would like to go for a walk.

Some people are early birds and want to get out and walk as the sun is just coming up.

Others prefer to walk in the cool air of the evening, right when the sun is beginning to go down.

Whatever time you choose to walk, you should make it consistent. By choosing a consistent time to walk each day or every other day, your body and mind will become accustomed to the physical exertion it will be required to engage in as you put your biological machine in motion. Before you begin walking, you should give thought to the route you will follow and the distance you will travel. These two things are extremely important.

Depending on your age, body weight composition, and physical ability, you should design a walking program that allows you to engage in this mild physical activity while remaining within your physical abilities and limitations.

If you are uncertain of your physical abilities, I would recommend starting with half a mile as a beginning point, and then build upon this as your strength, stamina, and physical conditioning grows stronger.

NOTE: It is estimated that the average person can burn approximately 100 calories during a one mile walk.

CHAPTER 14

RUNNING

If you like being outside in nature, then running is for you. When I was in Navy boot camp and the Los Angeles Police Academy, we did a lot of running. Running is a good exercise. If you have prior experience with running, such as in junior high school, high school, college athletics, or military training, then you should use what you learned in these institutions to guide you in the development of your own fitness regime. However, if you have no prior experience in the area of running, then I'd recommend you look up a few YouTube videos (after consulting a licensed physician), or maybe a health and fitness magazine or article that covers running, which can help you develop a beginner's program that suits you and your athletic needs.

CHAPTER 15

WALKING THE DOG

Walking your dog is an excellent exercise. Much like humans, dogs need physical movement too. Dogs require daily exercise to live strong, healthy, and quality lives. By walking your dog, or your neighbor's dog, or a friend's dog, you end up killing two birds with one stone, because you provide exercise for both the dog and yourself.

Pick a good route through your neighborhood; one that takes you past the homes of the nice people who live on your street, and just start walking.

CHAPTER 16
CYCLING

If you own a bicycle (I highly recommend that you do), and you live within three to four miles or so from a local grocery or convenience store, and you need a small item to prepare a healthy meal, I would recommend you to ride your bike to the store instead of burning petrol fuel and helping in further polluting the air. By riding your bike, you are forcing the largest muscles of the body to do the majority of the work. You are using the quadriceps (the four front muscles in the upper thigh), the hamstrings (rear upper leg muscles), and the calves (lower muscle group) every time you ride a bike. You are also accelerating the heart muscle, which is the most important muscle of all, for an extended period of time.

If you enjoy riding a bike and prefer this exercise over walking or running, then you should develop a program that allows you to ride at least three days each week.

You can start out with a mile, and then begin to add distance as you develop muscular strength and endurance. Riding your bike will help you burn excess calories and build muscular strength in the legs and buttocks.

STATIONARY BIKES

As was stated in an earlier chapter of this book, I have two stationary bikes; one in my bedroom, and the other, a fold-up bike, in the formal dining room area.

The reason I have two is simple. The one in my bedroom is a large, heavy, recumbent bike, on which I can sit back and peddle at my leisure.

The fold-up bike, that is kept in an upright position, in the dining room, is about 50 pounds lighter, and can be easily moved to positions either inside or outside the home.

The reason I have stationary bikes inside the home in addition to the street bikes I have in my garage is because the stationary bikes allow me to cycle without leaving the confines of the residence.

I am an avid TV watcher – and I love movies, especially military movies.

The stationary bikes (especially the fold-up bike) allow me to turn on one of the TV's at home, select a channel or put on one of my favorite movies, and just peddle away.

Before you I know it, I have ridden ten-miles, with almost no effort.

ADMONITION: Get a stationary bike. You will thank me!

NOTE: Some sporting goods stores offer stationary bikes for as little as around $100.

CHAPTER 17
WEIGHT-LIFTING

If you elect to lift weights as a part of your fitness/weight loss program, I recommend a program that I was introduced to about 25 years ago, when I was trying to gain muscular strength in my effort to join L.A.P.D.'s Elite Metropolitan Division, and then hopefully the S.W.AT. (Special Weapons and Tactics) unit.

The program involves working only one basic muscle group per day for six days; then, after taking a one-day rest , you start all over again.

By working only one muscle group per day, you then give that group of fatigued muscles seven whole days to recover before taxing them again.

> Note: When we lift weights, we engage in resistance training. We provide the targeted muscle group(s) with the force of resistance while lifting.

As we lift heavier weights, the fiber within our muscles gets injured or slightly damaged. This damage is caused because the muscles are taxed beyond their previous lifting abilities. A biological component known as lactic acid is released by the injured muscle fiber. This release causes a pronounced sourness in the muscle group. This soreness is good because it is a clear indication that you have worked the targeted muscle group(s) to the point of exhaustion. As you give the injured muscle group a full seven days to recover, the muscle fiber starts to rebuild. This rebuilding is how our muscles get stronger and sometimes larger.

Here is how my workout routine goes:

- Day 1: Chest and triceps

- Day 2: Calves

- Day 3: Arms (biceps)

- Day 4: Legs (quadriceps and calves)

- Day 5: Back and shoulders

- Day 6: Legs (hamstrings and calves)

While using the appropriate amount of weight for each given exercise, I then do four sets of 10 repetitions for each exercise until the soreness sets it. By working only one muscle group per day, per workout, your workout becomes faster and much more focused and condensed.

I now look forward to my workouts because I know that by doing them, I am keeping my body finely tuned and ready for any task that might present itself through the course of the day.

Scientific studies: A number of scientific studies in the area of muscular development have repeatedly proven that a body that has been pushed to develop muscular growth becomes a veracious calorie burner. They look for ways to burn calories even while you're asleep.

Your body is your temple and your home; it is the physical and biological structure in which you live. Be kind to your body and take care of it. It's the only one you will ever have in this life.

> NOTE: I did not go into the specifics regarding how to lift weights targeting each of the body parts detailed above since this is a book about "No Meals After 6:00 P.M." If you are either curious or interested in learning how to lift weights, I strongly recommend that you either join a gym, hire a workout coach, or purchase a book that will instruct you regarding the proper manner in which to lift weights for overall health and fitness.

CHAPTER 18

ABDOMINAL EXERCISE

Abdominal exercises should be done at least three times a week. By doing them, your core will be strengthened. I recommend doing them on the same day in which you do your leg exercises.

> Note: If you have never done abdominal exercises (sit-ups and crunches), I strongly recommend you purchase a book for instructions, or hire a fitness instructor to assist you.

CHAPTER 19

GARDENING

If working out is not your thing, but gardening is, then get out your gardening gloves, an old pair of jeans, and prepare to get dirty for an hour every day or every other day.

Gardening is hard work. It is a labor of love. It requires the devote to give several hours to take care of rose gardens, flower gardens, vegetable gardens, the soil, and so on, till the hard work starts producing fruitful results. As you move around doing gardening on your hands and knees, you expend a lot of energy, this energy expenditure burns calories.

By getting down into the dirt two, three, or even four times each week, you are bending, kneeling, stretching, digging, and reaching with your body. You are no longer stagnant, dormant, or sedentary— you are exercising.

CHAPTER 20

HOUSEWORK

For those who have no interest in working out in gyms with weights, or engaging in running, gardening, and other physical activities that promote good health, there is always housework to resort to.

Housework is the simple act of cleaning the space you inhabit.

While I was in the United States Navy, sailors were required to perform a weekly cleaning action referred to as conducting a 'Field Day'. A Field Day is the act of cleaning your work area, barracks, room, ship, aircraft hangar, or the area of assignment in an effort to prepare it for an inspection later on by a team of Navy personnel assigned to ensure cleaning discipline.

When I separated from the Navy, I brought this concept home with me. Once every week, I conduct a Field Day at home. In doing this, I sweep, mop, vacuum, dust, and clean my entire residence. This action puts my body in motion for a full one to two hours each time I do it. While cleaning my home, I am putting my body in motion for an extended period of time. Therefore, I'm replacing sleeping, lounging around, and couch time with this unconventional form of exercise.

Therefore, if you have no desire to work out, but enjoy cleaning, this is a fantastic way to keep moving.

NOTE: If your house is clean (because you just did it yesterday), then clean the home of someone you love and care for. Clean the home of an elderly person who lacks your physical strength. Clean the home of a person who is infirmed, and would be grateful for your kindness and generosity.

CHAPTER 21

AMOUNT OF WEIGHT THAT CAN BE LOST PER WEEK

It is recommended by most medical professionals that dieters should engage in efforts that will allow them to lose between one to two pounds per week.

For those who are seriously overweight and have a strong desire to change that, a major reduction in your daily calorie intake may be necessary to achieve your goal.

A major calorie intake reduction might mean no longer eating things like bacon, eggs, ham, hash browns, or a buttered bread breakfast. A heavy lunch (2,000 calories or more) at your favorite restaurant or fast food establishment, or a 2,000 to 3,000-calorie dinner at home are things that will be off-limits too. You will have to tailor your diet in a way that gives you all the nutrients needed for healthy living.

If you are seriously overweight, you might need to resort to consuming below 1,200 to 1,500 calories a day.

QUESTION: How does one get his or her daily calorie intake down to 1,200 to 1,500 calories?

ANSWER: By proper food management and discipline.

QUESTION: What is proper food management? ANSWER: Proper food management is taking a hard, straightforward, and honest look at the food you consume each day, and engaging in steps to reduce the total calorie count of what you put into your body.

EXAMPLE OF CALORIE INTAKE ADJUSTMENT:

Instead of having a huge breakfast containing about 2,000 calories, start your daily calorie intake with a bowl of oatmeal, which contains 130 to 150 calories and almost no fat.

Then, instead of a heavy lunch, have a low-calorie healthy salad, a protein bar, or a protein shake.

Now we come to one of the most important meals of the day - dinner.

Most people are conditioned since childhood that dinner is the biggest, grandest, and most important meal of the day, which is why they go all out. They have heavy, calorie-laden meals because they feel they have earned it, perhaps because they worked hard at the job site, school, college, or had a heavy workout at the gym. They feel no guilt in loading up the dinner plate with all it can hold.

Well, I am here to tell you that if you are battling a weight problem, which is a direct result of a combination of overeating and almost no exercise, you must end this practice.

If you are serious about changing your body and improving your life, this gluttonous mealtime behavior needs to stop. Instead of having a calorie-heavy dinner, I suggest you to have something small, light, and healthy; something that the stomach can easily burn through and process, as it marches towards ketosis. By dramatically reducing the number of calories you ingest daily (starting with breakfast and ending with dinner), you are turning your body into a fat-burning machine.

> NOTE: You are marching in the direction of healthy living, and superb fitness. Your body will have no choice. Your body is a MACHINE; it can only burn or store the fatty materials you feed it.

CHAPTER 22

SWIMMING

Don't like weights, cycling, walking, doing housework, gardening, or running? Well, there is always water.

Swimming is one of the best aerobic exercises available to us. An hour of swimming each day or every other day will transform your body.

You will burn calories, tone flabby muscles, lose fat, and vastly improve your overall level of fitness.

Swimming is refreshing, low-impact, cool, and invigorating.

It works pretty much all of the major muscle groups of the body.

CHAPTER 23

YOGA

The fundamental purpose of yoga is to foster harmony in the body, mind, and environment.

Yoga professes a complete system of physical, mental, social, and spiritual development.

For generations, this philosophy was passed on from the master teacher to the student.

> NOTE: If you are interested in learning about yoga, I recommend that you hire an instructor to guide you through learning the mechanics of this exercise discipline.

CHAPTER 24
PILATES

Pilates is a method of exercise that consists of low-impact flexibility and muscular strength and endurance movement.

Pilates emphasizes proper postural alignment, core strength, and muscle balance.

Pilates is named after its creator, Joseph Pilates, who developed the exercises in the 1920s.

> NOTE: If you are interested in this exercise discipline, I recommend that you hire a personal trainer that specializes in this particular form of physical fitness and development.

CHAPTER 25

AEROBICS

Aerobics is a form of physical exercise that combines rhythmic aerobic exercise with stretching, and strength training routines with the goal of improving all elements of fitness (flexibility, muscular strength, and cardio-vascular fitness).

Many gyms offer a variety of aerobic classes.

> NOTE: If you are interested in doing aerobic exercises and are unsure about your abilities, it might be a good idea to invest in a class or hire a personal trainer.

CHAPTER 26

SELF-DEFENSE: (BOXING/MARTIAL ARTS)

In today's society, self-protection and personal safety are of prime importance.. You could find yourself in a situation where you might have to defend yourself, or someone you love. The time to learn how to do it isn't during the moment of crisis, but before such a situation crops up. All military personnel, and police officers, are given some form of either self-defense or hand-to-hand combat training.

Just because you as a civilian have never worn a uniform, does not mean you should not know how to defend yourself.

By learning self-defense, you begin to better understand how your body works. You begin to better understand what it was designed to do.

Self-defense training can be rigorous. To warm up in preparation for a training session, you must engage nearly all of the major muscle groups of the body. Then, after warming up, you use them as you practice how to defend yourself.

BURNING CALORIES:

While training (boxing, punching, kicking, wrestling), you are engaging in a lot of physical exertion. This concentrated, focused expenditure of energy burns a lot of calories.

PROFESSIONAL INSTRUCTION:

If you are not sure of how to adequately protect and defend yourself from a potential aggressor, I strongly recommend that you invest financial resources, time, and effort in learning self-defense.

There are martial arts schools in nearly every city nowadays.

Go online, research which form of self-defense most suits your personal needs, and start moving in that direction. Help develop your overall physical conditioning and wellbeing.

Learn how to defend yourself!

CHAPTER 27

MUSCLE AND BONE DENSITY LOSS DUE TO A LACK OF EXERCISE

A number of studies have demonstrated scientifically that prolonged lazy or sedentary lifestyles contribute to the loss of both muscular strength and bone density.

People who live a sedentary lifestyle are destroying their own bodies through inactivity.

By sitting on the couch or lying in bed for hours every day, we deprive our bodies of motion, effort, and resistance. These actions are extremely detrimental to our health and overall fitness.

Our bodies were designed for motion. By failing to move for long periods of time and failing to provide resistance, the muscular structures of our skeletal systems begin to atrophy.

Like muscle, bone is a living tissue. This tissue requires physical activity to be healthy.

When astronauts spend long periods of time without resistance because of zero gravity during space travel, one of the many concerns for their physical well-being is loss of bone density and muscular atrophy.

Doctors, physical therapists, and others in the medical field all recommend physical activity and resistance training to counter muscular atrophy and loss of bone density.

CHAPTER 28

WATER

Water is an essential element of safe and healthy dieting. By drinking water, we help our body to both process and remove unwanted elements from within our systems.

It is recommended that we drink at least one glass of water a half an hour prior to consuming a meal, because this helps in filling up the stomach. By filling space in the stomach prior to eating a meal, you will eat less food, which will lead to the consumption of lesser calories.

I encourage all of those who I train in physical fitness in my home to drink water.

Bottles of water should be stored in your home as well as your workplace. When the urge hits for a quick food fix of junk food, causing you to momentarily move away from your goal of maintaining a healthy, nutritious diet routine, I want you to instead reach for one of those bottles of water. I want you to walk back from your home, office, or workplace refrigerator with a fresh bottle of water as a measure to satisfy the momentary craving.

CHAPTER 29

HEALTHY MEALS

Healthy meals are those that contain the highest nutritional value while having the lowest percentage of calories and fat.

Healthy meals should be thought out and planned beforehand. In fact, prior to going to the grocery store, you should be thinking about buying healthy food products that will lead to the making of healthy meals.

Healthy meals are well-balanced. They contain protein, fiber, and other nutrients and vitamins that our bodies require to function as designed.

If you are not accustomed to planning, cooking, or preparing healthy meals, there are a number of books and information online that can provide invaluable assistance to you in your efforts to live a healthier, fitter, and more prosperous lifestyle.

CHAPTER 30

PROTEIN SHAKES

Protein shakes are an excellent way to assist in your efforts to engage in the restriction of calorie intake.

Humans gain weight for two basic reasons:

1. We take in too many calories.

2. We don't burn enough of the calories we take in.

As a United States Navy Sailor, policeman, and police sergeant, I learned that one of the most important aspects of weight management is proper food intake.

By taking in too much food, you will gain weight over time if the calories aren't burned away. While working as a police officer, I found that I could both take in the proper amount of protein (for muscle building and muscular growth) and manage the amount of weight I gained by using protein shakes and protein bars.

The average protein shake contains roughly between 120 to 130 calories and almost zero fat. They typically contain only one percent carbohydrates and roughly 25 grams of protein.

By drinking a protein shake every three hours, you kill the craving for junk food and other undesirable substances that are not in line with your weight loss objectives.

You annihilate it!

In between your breakfast meal, when you break your 15-hour fast, and the last meal you have before 6:00 P.M., you are providing your body with the nutrients it needs to be fit and healthy while you maintain caloric intake discipline.

CHAPTER 31

DIET SPONSOR

In this chapter, I have elected to address an issue that plagues many people - the issue of addiction.

Millions of people all over the world suffer from addiction. People are addicted to drugs, alcohol, gambling, shopping, and yes – even food.

Addicts live with an unseen monster, a demon. It is an evil that does not love or care about you or your wellbeing. Addiction is not your friend; in fact, it is your worst enemy.

When we do things that bring us pleasure, like excessive shopping, gambling away the rent or mortgage money, using illegal (or even legal) drugs until we are comatose, or eating an entire extra-large pizza by ourselves, we give in to this demon. You are actively participating in the feeding of your addiction.

When we do things we enjoy, the brain rewards us with the release of a chemical called dopamine. Dopamine is a reward system that can lead us into a hellish existence.

We know that we desperately need to do something about being overweight, but because eating an entire gallon of ice cream and a full bag of potato chips causes a release of dopamine, we do it despite the consequences. If as you read this section of the book, it causes you to reel in horror because I am describing your behavior, you may be an addict. An addict hopelessly and desperately addicted to the excessive consumption of food.

If this chapter of the book has caused you to ask yourself this question, then you probably are.

RESOLUTION:

If the bathroom scale tells you that you are suffering from obesity or morbid obesity, it is time to do something about it. I want you take the following actions.

1. I want you to be honest with yourself that you are overweight.

2. I want you to admit to yourself that you may need help to resolve this food intake problem.

3. I want you to confide in someone who loves and cares about you that you have reached this conclusion.

4. I want you reach out for profession help from a diet doctor, a therapist, or a weight-management counselor.

5. I want you to start moving in a new direction; a direction of health, fitness, and self-love.

DIET SPONSOR:

In the world of addiction, many people have what is known as a sponsor. A sponsor is typically a person who has already fought and won the battle you are currently dealing with.

A sponsor is someone you can call when you are about to use the food delivery app on your phone at 9:00 P.M., to order a 3,000 calorie meal to be delivered to your home, because you are depressed and lonely and want to use food to make it all better. A sponsor is someone you can call while you're in the grocery store's pastry section, and you push your shopping cart past your favorite chocolate cake, and the demons that live in your brain command you to purchase it. A sponsor is the person who can help you re-focus and re-center you when you are about to make unhealthy food decisions.

A sponsor can keep you on the path to good health and good living.

A sponsor is someone who cares about you and loves you and wants to see you become your best self.

A sponsor can be a friend, a neighbor, a relative, or a professional person who has experience in dealing with this type of addiction.

CHAPTER 32

GARBAGE FOOD PURGE

QUESTION: What is garbage food?

ANSWER: Garbage food is any food that does not contribute to your overall health, fitness, and wellbeing.

Garbage food is what we eat when we are bored, depressed, lonely, or "fidgeting," and just want to do something with our hands and mouth.

Garbage food is the second candy bar; garbage food is opening a bag of potato chips or other kinds of hand food that comes in a bag. The information on the bag's exterior tells you that the bag contains 10 servings, at 250 calories per serving, and you consume (eat) the entire bag—all by yourself.

Garbage food is the stuff we eat when we are not hungry, but we consume them anyways because we have nothing else to do, or we are having cravings for junk food, or we open the food delivery app on our phone and order pizza, and hamburgers and fries, and other things we know we should not be consuming because we are engaged in the battle for overall good health and fitness.

THE PURGE:

If you are overweight and you sincerely want to change your life, I want you to go through your kitchen and even your bedroom if needed, and remove anything from within your home that tempts you; be it bags of candy, potato chips, ice cream, dips, pastries, cakes, pies, and any other food that calls to you and makes you weak while pursuing your fitness goal. The reason I want you to purge these items from your home is because most of us have difficulty resisting urges. When the urge hits, you tell yourself that you're just going to have one single scoop of ice cream, or just one slice of apple pie or one candy from the big bag. Just a few chips from a family-size bag.

Then, an hour or so later, you're disgusted with yourself. You hate yourself for eating not one slice of apple pie, but three. Not just one donut, but four. Not just a few pieces of candy from the family pack, but nearly one-third of it.

This is why I want you to go on a total purge of any and all junk food that may tempt you when you are weak.

CHAPTER 33

DIET PANIC

As you begin to change your eating habits by deciding to consume no food after 6:00 P.M. until 9:00 A.M., your mind and body will enter a kind of shock in the early days. Fasting for 15 hours will be foreign to both your mind and your body. The habits you have established over the years of your life—your body will remember. This is where personal discipline, determination, and the maturity factor kick in.

At some point, you will have to make the adult decision that adhering to the plan that will most assuredly allow you to reach your goal is far more important than consuming food after 6:00 P.M.

You will have to make the decision to not go searching in your refrigerator for mid-day, or late night snacks, and reach for a bottle of water instead. You will have to make the decision that you can indeed wait till cheat day to consume the food you love to eat like pizza, spaghetti and meatballs, roast beef, hamburgers, burritos, pie, cake, ice cream, and all the other things. However, if you are willing to maintain discipline by continuing to make mature and intelligent dietary decisions, this program can and will change your life.

QUESTION: How do I know this?

ANSWER: Because I went through all you are about to endure. This new way of thinking, this new way of living, this new way of deciding, helped me to lose nearly 40 pounds of unwanted, excess fat in just under seven months, with no surgeries or doctors or fitness instructors involved. If I can do it, then you can do it too!

EPILOGUE

It is my sincere hope that by purchasing and reading this book, you have made a decision that will have a positive and lasting impact on your life.

By incorporating discipline, intelligence, maturity, and a sincere desire to change, you can bring-out the real you.

If you elect to follow the dieting principles laid out in this little book, your body will change, and so will your life.

As we say in the United States Navy, *"Fair Winds and Following Seas."* Good luck to you.

Matthew: 6:10